Hormones and Breast Cancer

A Guide to Oestrogen's Role and Prevention

Sophia Royce Smartwell

DEDICATION

To all the courageous people impacted by breast cancer: we are always inspired by your fortitude and tenacity.

Many people's lives are being significantly improved by the researchers and medical professionals who are working nonstop to increase our knowledge of this illness and enhance available treatments.

And to the friends and family who never waver your encouragement and love are crucial on the path to recovery and hope.

You should read this book.

DISCLAIMER

Hormones and Breast Cancer: A Guide to Oestrogen's Role and Prevention contains information that is meant primarily for educational purposes and should not be used in place of expert medical advice, diagnosis, or treatment. If you have any questions about a medical condition or treatment, you should always consult your doctor or another trained healthcare professional.

Regarding the correctness, completeness, and dependability of the information in this book, the publishers and authors offer no guarantees or assurances. Before making any adjustments to your treatment plan or regimen, it is crucial to speak with a knowledgeable healthcare practitioner because individual health problems and circumstances might differ significantly.

By using this book, you understand and accept that the publishers and authors cannot be held accountable for any negative outcomes or repercussions that may arise from applying or using any of the material in it.

CONTENTS

ACKNOWLEDGMENTS...

CHAPTER 1...

Breast Cancer Overview...

    1.1. Breast Cancer Overview...

    1.2. Breast Cancer Types... 2

    1.3. Important Breast Cancer Risk Factors................................. 5

CHAPTER 2... 10

Hormones' Contribution to Breast Cancer.................................. 10

    2.1. Overview of Hormonal Factors in the Development of Cancer.... 10

    2.2. Summary of the Function of Estrogen in the Body...................... 11

    2.3. The Impact of Estrogen on Breast Tissue and the Development of Cancer.. 13

CHAPTER 3... 19

Breast Cancer and Oestrogen Receptors.................................. 19

    3.1. Breast cancer that is ER+ (estrogen receptor-positive)................ 19

    3.2. How Tumor Growth Is Caused by Oestrogen Receptor Activation.. 21

    3.3. Oestrogen Receptor Status Testing....................................... 24

CHAPTER 4... 28

Risk of Breast Cancer and Oestrogen Metabolism......................... 28

    4.1. Summary of the Body's Estrogen Metabolism............................ 28

    4.2. Metabolic Pathways' Impact on Cancer Risk............................ 30

    4.3. Estrogen Metabolism Genetic Factors..................................... 33

CHAPTER 5... 37

The Risk of Breast Cancer and Hormone Replacement Therapy (HRT) 37

5.1. Hormone Replacement Treatment Types.................................37

5.2. How Breast Cancer Risk Is Increased by HRT..............................39

5.3. Recommendations for HRT Safety................................. 43

CHAPTER 6...48

Treatment of Breast Cancer with Oestrogen Blockers...........................48

6.1. Estrogen Blockers' Mode of Action................................48

6.2. Tamoxifen: An ER+ Breast Cancer Standard Treatment..............50

6.3. Novel Treatments for Estrogen Blocking............................. 53

CHAPTER 7...58

The Function of Aromatase Inhibitors in Breast Cancer......................58

7.1. Aromatase Inhibitors: What Are They?.............................58

7.2. Aromatase's Function in Postmenopausal Estrogen Production....59

7.3. A Comparison of Oestrogen Blockers and Aromatase Inhibitors. 61

CHAPTER 8...66

Lifestyle and Environmental Aspects Affecting Estrogen Levels......... 66

8.1. Diet and How It Affects Oestrogen Production............................66

8.2. Obesity and Elevated Production of Oestrogen.............................69

8.3. Estrogen Disruption and Environmental Toxins...........................72

CHAPTER 9...76

Strategies to Prevent Breast Cancer Caused by Oestrogen...................76

9.1. The Significance of Prompt Identification in Cancers Associated with Oestrogen...76

9.2: Does Prophylactic Oestrogen Suppression Work?.......................79

9.3 Changes in Lifestyle to Reduce Estrogen Levels........................... 8

CHAPTER 10...**8**

Research on Breast Cancer and Oestrogen Targeting in the Future....8

10.1. Advances in ER+ Breast Cancer Targeted Therapies.................. 8

10.2. Genetic Studies of Mutations in Estrogen Receptors................. 9

10.3. Oestrogen Profile-Based Customized Treatment Plans.............. 9

ABOUT THE AUTHOR..**9**

ACKNOWLEDGMENTS

My sincere appreciation goes out to everyone who helped with ***Hormones and Breast Cancer: A Guide to Oestrogen's Role and Prevention.***

I want to start by expressing my gratitude to the brave people who have battled breast cancer. My comprehension of this illness has been greatly influenced by your tales and experiences, which have also motivated me to provide knowledge that could help others on their path.

My sincere gratitude goes out to the medical personnel and researchers whose unwavering commitment to breast cancer research served as the basis for this publication. Your discoveries and insights have shed light on the intricate relationship between hormones and breast cancer, allowing others to gain knowledge and experience from your knowledge.

I would especially like to thank my friends and family for their constant encouragement and support during this undertaking. Your confidence in me inspired me to write and served as a constant reminder of how important it is to spread this important knowledge.

I want to express my gratitude to my editors and reviewers for their insightful criticism and help in improving the material. Your knowledge made it possible for people of different backgrounds to enjoy this book in addition to its educational value.

Lastly, I want to thank everyone who has read this book. It is admirable how dedicated you are to study more about estrogen and breast cancer. As you traverse this crucial area of health and wellness, I hope this book proves to be a useful tool.

I appreciate everyone's participation in this adventure.

CHAPTER 1

BREAST CANCER OVERVIEW

1.1. Breast Cancer Overview

Although it can also strike men, breast cancer is one of the most prevalent malignancies in the world to harm women. It starts in the breast cells, usually in the lobules (which generate milk) or ducts (which transport milk to the nipple). Cells in the breast tissue change abnormally in breast cancer, expanding out of control to form tumors. While some tumors are malignant (cancerous), which means they can spread to other parts of the body via the lymphatic or circulatory systems, others are benign (non-cancerous).

Breast cancer is classified according to its behavior and place of origin. The prognosis is considerably improved by early identification and intervention. Every year, more than 2 million new cases of breast cancer are detected, according to the World Health Organization (WHO). Awareness, early identification, and research into prevention and therapy are crucial since, despite breakthroughs in treatment, breast cancer continues to be the primary cause of cancer-related death among women.

Important information on breast cancer:

Affecting millions of women globally, the prevalence varies according to socioeconomic and geographic circumstances.

Breast lumps, changes in breast size or shape, nipple discharge, or changes in breast skin are examples of common symptoms.

Early-stage (breast-only) and advanced-stage (metastatic cancer spreading to other organs) are the two stages of development.

1.2. Breast Cancer Types

Breast cancer has multiple subtypes, each with unique

traits and treatment consequences, rather than being a single illness. Determining the best course of treatment requires an understanding of the many forms of breast cancer. In general, there are two forms of breast cancer: invasive and non-invasive (in situ).

The non-invasive breast cancer known as "ductal carcinoma in situ" (DCIS) is characterized by aberrant cells that are limited to the milk ducts and have not yet migrated to neighboring tissues. With the right care, DCIS, an early kind of breast cancer, has a good chance of being cured.

About 80% of instances of breast cancer are of the most prevalent kind, invasive ductal carcinoma (IDC). Although IDC starts in the milk ducts, it can spread to other parts of the body by invading adjacent breast tissue.

ILC, or invasive lobular carcinoma, is: Less often than IDC, this kind starts in the lobules. ILC frequently manifests as a mild breast thickening, which makes it more difficult to identify during physical examinations or mammograms.

The aggressive kind of breast cancer known as triple-negative breast cancer (TNBC) is insensitive to several of the most popular hormonal treatments because it lacks HER2 receptors, progesterone, and estrogen. Compared to other forms, TNBC typically grows more quickly and has a higher likelihood of recurring.

Positive Breast Cancer for HER2: The overexpression of the HER2 protein, which stimulates the growth of cancer cells, is what distinguishes this variety. In order to improve the prognosis of patients with HER2-positive cancer, targeted medicines such as trastuzumab (Herceptin) have been developed to prevent the action of this protein.

Hormone Receptor-Positive Breast Cancer: Breast cancers that express progesterone or estrogen receptors (ER/PR-positive) are more likely to respond favorably to hormonal therapy that deactivate the hormones' growth-promoting effects. Compared to some other forms, hormone receptor-positive tumors typically grow more slowly and have better prognosis.

One to five percent of all occurrences of breast cancer are inflammatory breast cancer (IBC), an uncommon but severe type of the disease. Usually without a noticeable lump, it manifests as breast warmth, redness, and swelling. IBC spreads and grows quickly, therefore increasing survival rates requires early identification.

Breast Paget's Disease: This uncommon kind of cancer affects the areola and nipple skin. It frequently coexists with underlying breast cancer, either invasive or DCIS, and manifests as nipple crusting, scaling, or bleeding.

Because the biology of cancer affects therapy options and results, it is crucial to comprehend these subtypes. As scientists learn more about the molecular and genetic variations among these subtypes, precision medicine techniques which customize treatment to the unique features of the tumor are proliferating.

1.3. Important Breast Cancer Risk Factors

Although the precise origin of breast cancer is still

unknown, there are a number of risk factors that ar associated with a higher chance of getting the disease These elements fall into two groups: modifiable an non-modifiable.

Risk factors that cannot be changed:

- **Gender:** The biggest risk element is being a woman Breast cancer is approximately 100 times more common in women than in males, despite the fact that it can occur in men.

- **Age:** As people age, especially after the age of fifty, their risk of developing breast cancer rises. Women over 55 are diagnosed with the majority of breast cancer cases.

- **Genetic Mutations:** The risk of ovarian and breast cancers is greatly increased by inherited mutations in the BRCA1 and BRCA2 genes. The risk may also be increased by additional genetic alterations, such as those in the TP53 or CHEK2 genes.

- **Family History:** If a woman has close family members (mother, sister, or daughter) who have had breast cancer, especially when they were young, her risk is increased. Hereditary breast cancer accounts for 5–10% of cases.

- **Personal History of Breast Cancer:** Women who have previously experienced breast cancer are more likely to experience it again, either in the same breast or a different one.

- **Race and Ethnicity:** African American women are more likely to die from breast cancer because of variables like more aggressive tumor forms and unequal access to care, while white women are slightly more likely to have the disease than Asian, Hispanic, or African American women.

The following are modifiable risk factors:

- **Reproductive History:** A woman's exposure to estrogen is increased during early menstruation (before the age of 12) and late menopause (beyond the age of 55), and this is associated with an increased risk of breast cancer. Risk is also increased by not having children at all or by having the first full-term pregnancy after the age of thirty.

- **Hormone Replacement Therapy (HRT)**: Following menopause, prolonged usage of a combination of estrogen and progesterone hormone therapy is linked to a higher risk of breast cancer.

- **Alcohol Consumption:** Studies indicate that women who drink alcohol have an increased risk of breast cancer, and the risk rises as alcohol intake does.

- **Obesity and Lack of Physical Activity:** Being overweight raises the risk of breast cancer because excess adipose tissue produces more estrogen, especially after menopause. Another established risk factor is a sedentary lifestyle.

- **Radiation Exposure:** Women who had radiation therapy to the chest as children or adolescents for another cancer (such Hodgkin's lymphoma) are more likely to get breast cancer in the future.

- **Diet and Nutrition:** Although studies are still being conducted, some indicate that a diet heavy in processed foods and saturated fats may raise the risk of breast cancer.

Strategies for early detection and prevention both depend on an understanding of these risk factors. In order to determine their risk and investigate preventive options like lifestyle modifications or prophylactic surgery, women who are more susceptible owing to family history or genetic predispositions can have more regular testing or genetic counseling.

Adopting good lifestyle practices, remaining aware of one's own risk, and getting frequent tests can significantly lower the chance of developing breast cancer, even when some risk factors are out of an individual's control.

CHAPTER 2

HORMONES' CONTRIBUTION TO BREAST CANCER

2.1. Overview of Hormonal Factors in the Development of Cancer

Growth, metabolism, and reproduction are just a few of the biological processes that hormones regulate. The relationship between hormones and cellular activity is especially important in the setting of breast cancer. Because breast tissue is hormonally responsive, both normal breast development and the aberrant growth of malignant cells have been related to specific hormones, most notably estrogen and progesterone.

The presence of hormone receptors on cancer cells is a common way to classify breast cancer. These receptors enable the usage of progesterone and estrogen by cancer cells to support their development. Hormone receptor-positive cancers are those that express these hormone receptors, whereas hormone receptor-negative cancers do not. A significant percentage of breast cancer patients are hormone receptor-positive, particularly estrogen receptor-positive (ER-positive) forms, which are responsive to hormone-blocking treatments.

Hormones have a complex and multifaceted impact on the development of breast cancer. In summary, by attaching itself to particular receptors, estrogen can stimulate the growth of breast cells, even malignant ones. Because of this, knowing hormonal pathways is essential for creating preventative and therapeutic plans. The relationship between hormones and breast cancer emphasizes how crucial hormone management is to the treatment of the condition. The mainstay of treatment for breast cancer, particularly for tumors that are hormone receptor-positive, is hormone therapy, which either inhibits the effects of estrogen or lowers its production.

2.2. Summary of the Function of Estrogen in the Body

One essential hormone that is essential to the growth and operation of the female reproductive system is estrogen. It controls a number of bodily functions, such as menstruation, pregnancy, menopause, and puberty. Although the ovaries create the majority of estrogen, minor amounts are also made in adipose tissue and the adrenal glands, particularly after menopause.

Estrogen is essential for women's reproductive tissues such as the ovaries, uterus, and breasts, to remain healthy. In addition to reproduction, estrogen plays important roles in:

1. **Bone health:** By regulating the loss and regrowth of bone tissue, estrogen contributes to the maintenance of bone density. An elevated risk of osteoporosis may result from a decrease in estrogen levels, which occurs following menopause.

2. **Cardiovascular health:** It is thought that estrogen protects the heart by raising HDL (good cholesterol) and lowering LDL (bad cholesterol), though this effect wears off after menopause.

3. Hormonal changes can have an effect on mental health since estrogen affects mood control, cognitive abilities, and even the protection of brain cells.

Estrogen levels vary during a woman's menstrual cycle. Estrogen levels increase during the follicular phase, the first half of the cycle, which promotes the development of the uterine lining in anticipation of a potential pregnancy. Just before ovulation, estrogen levels reach their highest, and if pregnancy is not achieved, they progressively decline. In addition to being a normal component of a woman's hormone cycle, these cyclical oscillations highlight how sensitive breast tissue is to hormonal shifts, which can affect the risk of cancer.

Estrogen still plays a part in postmenopausal women, but at a reduced level. The main source of estrogen is fat tissue, which produces it by converting androgens, or male hormones, into estrogen. This clarifies why a higher risk of post-menopausal breast cancer is linked to obesity, which increases fat tissue.

2.3. The Impact of Estrogen on Breast Tissue and the Development of Cancer

Since estrogen regulates both normal development and aberrant cell proliferation, its effects on breast tissue are complex. Estrogen promotes the development of breast ducts and lobules throughout puberty, which aids in the maturation of breast tissue. The development of sexuality and reproductive function depend on this natural and necessary process. But when this same capacity to encourage cell division and expansion feeds the unchecked growth of cancer cells, it can become troublesome.

Estrogen Receptors and Cancer Growth: The surface of many breast cancer cells has estrogen receptors (ER). Estrogen triggers signals that lead to the growth and division of cancer cells when it attaches to these receptors. Similar to how estrogen encourages the growth of healthy breast cells, this process turns harmful when cancer cells take advantage of it. Estrogen is a vital target for treatment since ER-positive breast tumors, which account for roughly 70% of all occurrences of breast cancer, thrive on it.

Breast cancer with hormone replacement therapy (HRT): By raising estrogen levels, hormone replacement therapy is frequently used to treat menopausal symptoms. However, prolonged use of this treatment has been associated with an increased risk of breast cancer. Because combined estrogen-progesterone therapy continuously stimulates breast tissue, which may result in malignant alterations, it has a higher risk of breast cancer than estrogen-only therapy. HRT should therefore be carefully examined, particularly in women who have other breast cancer risk factors.

Proliferation and Mutation: In addition to promoting breast cell proliferation, estrogen may also have an impact on the emergence of genetic mutations that result in cancer. Oxidative stress is brought on by reactive oxygen species (ROS), which are produced by the body's metabolism of estrogen. Because of the potential for DNA damage from this oxidative stress, there is a greater chance of mutations that aid in the development and spread of breast cancer. Consequently, estrogen contributes to the mutagenesis environment that supports the formation of malignant cells in addition to acting as a growth factor.

Carcinogenic Risk and Estrogen Metabolism: Breast cancer risk may be influenced by the body's metabolism of estrogen. Different metabolites of estrogen are produced, and some of these have been found to have more potent carcinogenic effects than others. For instance 2-hydroxyestrone is believed to be more protective against breast cancer, whereas the metabolite 16α-hydroxyestrone has been associated with an increased risk of the disease. Both genetic and environmental variables influence the equilibrium of these metabolites, indicating that metabolism is a key element in the development of breast cancer.

Postmenopausal Breast Cancer and Estrogen: Peripheral adipose tissue, not the ovaries, is the main source of estrogen in postmenopausal women. In these fat cells, androgens are converted into estrogen by the enzyme aromatase. As a result, women who have more body fat, particularly belly fat may also produce more estrogen, which can encourage the development of breast tumors that are hormone receptor-positive. This explains why obesity is a major risk factor for postmenopausal women's breast cancer.

Targeted medicines: Because estrogen has been linked to breast cancer, targeted medicines that either inhibit its effects or lower the body's production of it have been developed. These treatments consist of:

- Tamoxifen and other medications known as selective estrogen receptor modulators (SERMs) attach to the estrogen receptors on breast cancer cells and stop estrogen from activating them. Tamoxifen is frequently used to treat and prevent breast cancer that is ER-positive.

- The enzyme aromatase, which converts androgens to estrogen, is blocked by medications such as letrozole and anastrozole for postmenopausal women. Hormone receptor-positive cancers are deprived of the estrogen they require to proliferate as a result of the decrease in estrogen levels.

- The risk of breast cancer recurrence in ER-positive cases can be decreased by drastically lowering estrogen levels in premenopausal women by inhibiting ovarian function by surgery or medication.

Estrogen contributes to the normal growth of breast tissue as well as the advancement of some forms of breast cancer. Many patients' fates have improved dramatically as a result of successful treatments that target hormone receptor-positive tumors, made possible by a better understanding of estrogen's molecular effects on breast tissue. A vital component of breast cancer prevention and treatment is hormonal regulation, which can be achieved through both pharmacological and lifestyle changes.

CHAPTER 3

BREAST CANCER AND OESTROGEN RECEPTORS

3.1. Breast cancer that is ER+ (estrogen receptor-positive)

A subtype of breast cancer known as estrogen receptor-positive (ER+) breast cancer is identified by the expression of estrogen receptors on the cell surface. These receptors enable the cancer cells to react to estrogen, which promotes the proliferation of the cells. About 70–80% of instances of breast cancer are ER+ breast cancer, which is the most prevalent kind, especially in postmenopausal women. These receptors' presence affects the prognosis and available treatments in addition to defining the features of the cancer.

ER+ breast cancers typically have a better prognosis since they develop more slowly than their ER-negative counterparts. However, because these cancers depend on

estrogen, excessive estrogen levels can either support o
worsen their growth. Because it addresses the cancer'
reliance on estrogen to stop its progression and recurrence
hormone therapy becomes a vital component of treatment.

Using hormone therapy that either blocks the estroger
receptors on cancer cells or lower the body's production o
estrogen is one of the most important parts of treating ER+
breast cancer. Selective Estrogen Receptor Modulators
(SERMs), such as tamoxifen, are among these treatments;
they attach to estrogen receptors and prevent estrogen from
activating them. In postmenopausal women, aromatase
inhibitors (AIs), such letrozole and anastrozole, are
frequently used to inhibit the enzyme aromatase, which
changes androgens into estrogen, hence reducing the
body's levels of estrogen. Patients with ER+ breast cancer
now have much higher survival rates thanks to these
hormone treatments.

In general, ER+ breast cancer has a favorable prognosis,
particularly if caught early. Recurrence risk is still an issue,
though, and patients may need long-term hormone therapy
to lower the chance of the cancer coming back.

Additionally, over time, ER+ breast cancer may become resistant to hormone therapy, making treatment more difficult and requiring more research into causes of resistance.

3.2. How Tumor Growth Is Caused by Oestrogen Receptor Activation

One of the main factors influencing the development and spread of ER+ breast cancer is estrogen receptor activation. A series of biochemical processes inside the cell are set off when estrogen attaches to its receptor (ER), which results in tumor growth and cell division. The majority of this receptor-ligand interaction takes place in the cancer cell's nucleus, where the estrogen-receptor complex acts as a transcription factor to control the production of genes essential for cell survival and proliferation.

- **Mechanism of Action:** When estrogen attaches itself to the estrogen receptor, the receptor changes shape, enabling dimerization, or pairing with another estrogen receptor. After entering the cell's nucleus, this estrogen-ER complex attaches itself to particular

DNA sequences called estrogen response elements (EREs). The transcription of genes that support cell division and growth is started when this complex binds to EREs. As the cell cycle progresses from the G1 phase to the S phase, where DNA replication takes place, several of these genes are involved.

- **Downstream Effects:** These genes' activation increases cell proliferation while also blocking apoptotic pathways, which makes it less likely that cancer cells would naturally die off. Tumor growth results from a net rise in the number of cancer cells. Growth factors like insulin-like growth factor (IGF-1) and genes involved in cell cycle regulation, such Cyclin D1, are among the important genes controlled by estrogen signaling.

- **Cross-talk with Other Pathways:** Activation of the estrogen receptor may also have an impact on other cellular signaling pathways, including those involving cytokines and growth factors. For instance, the PI3K/AKT and MAPK pathways, which are both implicated in cell growth and survival, are known to be influenced by estrogen receptor signaling. Tumor growth is further aided by this cross-talk, which intensifies the cancer cell's proliferative signals. Furthermore, the estrogen receptor has the ability to trigger non-genomic signaling cascades that occur outside of the nucleus which can encourage quick cellular reactions that aid in the development and spread of tumors.

- **Resistance Mechanisms:** Regretfully, over time, certain ER+ breast tumors become resistant to hormone treatments. A number of processes, including changes in the estrogen receptor itself that enable it to function even in the absence of estrogen, can cause this resistance. Furthermore, the need for estrogen receptor activation may be circumvented by enhanced activation of other growth pathways, such as the PI3K/AKT or HER2 pathways, which would permit the cancer cells to proliferate in spite of hormone therapy. One of the main goals of current breast cancer research is to comprehend and overcome these resistance mechanisms.

3.3. Oestrogen Receptor Status Testing

An essential first step in the diagnosis and treatment o breast cancer is testing for the presence of the estroger receptor. Since hormone therapy only works on tumors tha express the estrogen receptor, knowing whether a breas cancer is ER+ or ER-negative aids in customizing treatment plans. A biopsy of the tumor tissue is used tc determine whether estrogen receptors are present, and the testing procedure usually entails the following steps:

1. **Immunohistochemistry (IHC):** The most popular technique for determining ER status. IHC testing involves treating a tumor tissue sample with antibodies that bind to the estrogen receptor specifically. Under a microscope, the tissue sample will change color as a result of the antibody binding if estrogen receptors are present. A pathologist next evaluates the percentage and intensity of stained cells to determine whether the tumor is ER-positive. If at least 1% of the cancer cells stain for the estrogen receptor, the tumor is usually classified as

ER+.

2. **Scoring ER Status:** The percentage of cancer cells that tested positive for the estrogen receptor is often displayed in the IHC test findings. The percentage of cells having detectable ER expression is represented by a score ranging from 1 to 100%. Furthermore, the staining strength is frequently used to determine an intensity score, which ranges from 0 to 3. When combined, these values give a general idea of the tumor's estrogen receptor content and likelihood of responding to hormone treatment.

3. **Decisions Regarding Treatment and ER Status:** When choosing a course of treatment, knowing one's ER status is essential. Hormone treatments that either decrease estrogen synthesis (such as aromatase inhibitors) or block the estrogen receptor (such as tamoxifen) are commonly used to treat ER+ malignancies. When detected early, these treatments are typically successful in reducing or halting the progression of ER+ malignancies. ER-negative tumors, on the other hand, do not react to hormone therapy since they do not depend on estrogen for growth. Depending on the tumor's other molecular

features, these malignancies might need different therapies like chemotherapy or targeted medicines.

4. **Additional Receptor Testing:** Progesterone receptor (PR) and human epidermal growth factor receptor 2 (HER2) status are also evaluated for breast cancer tumors in addition to estrogen receptor status. Oncologists can classify breast cancer into subtypes, such as hormone receptor-positive (ER+/PR+) or triple-negative (ER-/PR-/HER2-), and therapy planning is guided by the combination of ER, PR, and HER2 outcomes. Compared to tumors that are ER+ but PR-negative, those that are both ER and PR positive typically have a better prognosis and respond better to hormone treatments.

A prevalent and important subtype of breast cancer that depends on estrogen signaling for growth is estrogen receptor-positive breast cancer. Effective hormone therapies that target the estrogen receptor have been developed as a result of a better understanding of the mechanisms underlying estrogen receptor activation and how it contributes to tumor growth. By directing the use of hormone-based medicines in the fight against breast cancer, testing for estrogen receptor status is a crucial diagnostic step that influences treatment plans and enhances patient outcomes.

CHAPTER 4

RISK OF BREAST CANCER AND OESTROGEN METABOLISM

4.1. Summary of the Body's Estrogen Metabolism

The hormone estrogen is essential for controlling sexual development, reproductive function, and other physiological functions in both men and women. The ovaries create the majority of estrogen in women prior to menopause, and after menopause, it is also produced in peripheral organs such as fat cells and adrenal glands. The intricate biochemical mechanisms via which the body produces, uses, and degrades estrogen into active and inactive forms are collectively referred to as estrogen metabolism.

There are three main types of estrogen:

1. **Estrone (E1):** In postmenopausal women, this weak type of estrogen predominates.
2. The strongest and most prevalent estrogen in a

woman's reproductive years is **estradiol (E2).**

3. A weak form of estrogen that is mostly found during pregnancy is called **Estriol (E3).**

After being created, estrogen travels through the circulation and attaches itself to different cells' estrogen receptors to start working biologically. Estrogen must then be metabolized and eliminated by the body in order to preserve equilibrium and avoid excessive buildup. The primary mechanism by which estrogen is metabolized in the liver is called hydroxylation, which transforms estrogen into a variety of metabolites with distinct biological functions.

Hydroxylation mechanisms: There are two main mechanisms by which estrogen is converted into various hydroxylated forms:

1. Because of its poor estrogenic action, 2-hydroxyestrone (2-OHE1), which is produced by the **2-Hydroxylation Pathway,** is regarded as a "protective" metabolite.

2. A metabolite with substantial estrogenic action, 16α-hydroxyestrone (16α-OHE1), is produced by the

16α-Hydroxylation Pathway and has been associated with an increased risk of breast cancer because of its capacity to strongly stimulate cell proliferation.

3. The production of 4-hydroxyestrone (4-OHE1), another strong estrogen metabolite that can create reactive intermediates that can damage and mutate DNA, is accomplished by the **4-Hydroxylation Pathway.**

Whether estrogen's effects will favor cellular health or contribute to carcinogenesis depends critically on the balance between these metabolic pathways. These metabolites are subsequently conjugated (rendered water soluble) and eliminated by the kidneys or bile as estrogen is degraded. Any disruption in this metabolic process could result in extended exposure to active metabolites of estrogen, raising the chance of developing breast cancer.

4.2. Metabolic Pathways' Impact on Cancer Risk

The possible risk for breast cancer is greatly influenced by the metabolism of estrogen. Metabolism is a major factor in determining cancer risk because different metabolic pathways produce estrogen metabolites with different amounts of estrogenic activity and carcinogenic potential.

The 2-hydroxylation route produces estrogen metabolites, such as 2-hydroxyestrone (2-OHE1), which have limited estrogenic activity and are typically thought to have protective effects. These metabolites have been linked to a lower risk of breast cancer development and are less likely to promote the proliferation of breast cells. Healthy estrogen metabolism is frequently indicated by higher levels of 2-OHE1 relative to other metabolites.

Conversely, estrogen metabolites produced through the 4-hydroxylation and 16α-hydroxylation routes can have strong genotoxic or estrogenic effects.

A potent estrogenic substance that stimulates cell division, 16α-hydroxyestrone (16α-OHE1) has been connected to a higher risk of hormone-dependent malignancies, including endometrial and breast cancers. It is an important risk factor for breast cancer because of its capacity to increase estrogen signaling in breast tissue.

In addition to its estrogenic action, 4-hydroxyestrone

(4-OHE1) can be further metabolically converted into quinones, which are reactive substances that can directly harm DNA and produce mutations that could either cause or encourage the development of cancer. One important mechanism connecting this pathway to breast cancer risk is the creation of DNA adducts, which are segments of DNA attached to a chemical that causes cancer.

DNA Damage and the Estrogen-Quinone Pathway: Estrogen quinones can be created by further oxidizing the metabolites (4-OHE1 and 4-OHE2) that are produced when estrogen is broken down via the 4-hydroxylation route. These extremely reactive substances have the ability to create covalent connections with DNA, which results in the creation of DNA adducts. The accumulation of mutations can start carcinogenesis if the body's DNA repair systems are unable to effectively repair this damage. Because it highlights a direct method by which estrogen metabolism adds to the mutational burden linked to the development of breast cancer, this process is especially worrisome.

Hydroxyestrone to 16α-Hydroxyestrone Ratio: In investigations of breast cancer risk, researchers frequently look at the ratio of 2-OHE1 to 16α-OHE1. A decreased risk of breast cancer is linked to a larger 2:16 ratio, which indicates a greater relative generation of beneficial 2-hydroxyestrone versus dangerous 16α-hydroxyestrone. On the other hand, because it indicates increased estrogenic activity that stimulates tumor growth, a low 2:16 ratio is regarded as a risk factor for breast cancer.

4.3. Estrogen Metabolism Genetic Factors

Genetic differences are a major factor in defining an individual's estrogen metabolism and, in turn, their risk of breast cancer. The enzymes involved in the metabolism of estrogen are encoded by a number of genes, and mutations in these genes can result in variations in metabolic activity, which can affect the ratio of carcinogenic to protective metabolites.

The hydroxylation of estrogen is carried out by the enzymes CYP1A1 and CYP1B1. While CYP1B1 prefers the 4-hydroxylation pathway, which can result in toxic, DNA-damaging metabolites, CYP1A1 prefers the 2-hydroxylation pathway, which yields protective metabolites. These enzymes' activity and, thus, the equilibrium between these pathways might be impacted by genetic variations.

- Higher levels of 4-hydroxyestrone may be produced by people with genetic variations that increase CYP1B1 activity, raising their risk of breast cancer. On the other hand, increased CYP1A1 activity might promote the synthesis of protective 2-hydroxyestrone, which lowers the risk of cancer.

The important enzyme COMT (Catechol-O-Methyltransferase) helps neutralize the potentially hazardous estrogen metabolites (like 4-OHE1) by adding a methyl group, which reduces their reactivity. The body's capacity to detoxify these toxic estrogen metabolites may be hampered by variations in the COMT gene that result in decreased enzyme activity. Because they are more exposed to genotoxic estrogen metabolites, people with reduced COMT activity may be more susceptible to breast cancer.

Glutathione S-Transferase (GST) Genes: The detoxification of estrogen quinones, which are reactive substances that might harm DNA, is aided by GST enzymes. The body's capacity to neutralize these substances may be diminished by genetic variations in the GST gene, increasing oxidative stress and DNA damage in breast tissue. Breast cancer may develop and spread as a result of this elevated genotoxic burden.

Uridine Diphosphate Glucuronosyltransferase (UGT) and Sulfotransferase (SULT) Genes: These enzymes are crucial for the conjugation and elimination of metabolites of estrogen. The rate at which estrogen and its byproducts are removed from the body can be impacted by variations in these genes. A higher risk of breast cancer may arise from extended exposure to active forms of estrogen due to impaired excretion of estrogen metabolites.

Polymorphisms of the estrogen receptor: Although the enzymes involved in estrogen metabolism are the main focus, genetic differences in the estrogen receptor genes (ESR1 and ESR2) may also affect the risk of breast cancer. The way that breast tissue reacts to estrogen can be influenced by polymorphisms in these receptors; certain variations have been connected to altered receptor activity or enhanced receptor sensitivity, which may raise the risk of breast cancer.

Customizing breast cancer preventive measures requires an understanding of the genetic factors influencing estrogen metabolism. Targeted interventions, such pharmaceutical treatments or lifestyle modifications, may help people with certain genetic predispositions alter their risk. By revealing a person's metabolic profile, genetic testing can help develop more individualized strategies for lowering the risk of breast cancer through dietary, environmental, and hormonal changes.

The balance of carcinogenic and beneficial metabolites in estrogen shapes the chance of tumor growth, making it a key factor in breast cancer risk. Genetic differences also affect how estrogen is detoxified and metabolized, which helps explain why some people are more vulnerable than others. New approaches to the prevention and treatment of breast cancer are constantly being made possible by our growing understanding of these processes.

CHAPTER 5

THE RISK OF BREAST CANCER AND HORMONE REPLACEMENT THERAPY (HRT)

5.1. Hormone Replacement Treatment Types

The main goal of hormone replacement therapy (HRT) is to relieve menopausal symptoms by restoring hormones that the body is no longer producing in sufficient quantities. HRT has been linked to a higher risk of breast cancer, despite the fact that it can be useful in treating menopausal symptoms such hot flashes, night sweats, vaginal dryness, and bone loss. The type of HRT, how long it is used for, and personal health considerations all affect the risk.

HRT comes in two primary varieties:

1. **Estrogen-Only HRT:** In this type of treatment, only estrogen is administered. Because estrogen alone can raise the risk of endometrial cancer without the balancing action of progesterone, it is usually

recommended to women who have had a hysterectomy (removal of the uterus). Compared to combined HRT, estrogen-only HRT is usually thought to carry a decreased risk of breast cancer.

2. **Combined HRT (Estrogen and Progesterone)** This kind of HRT lowers the risk of endometria cancer in women who still have their uterus by combining estrogen and progesterone (or a synthetic form called progestin). However, especially when used for an extended period of time, combined HRT has been more firmly linked to an elevated risk of breast cancer.

Additional types of hormone replacement therapy include:

1. **Bioidentical Hormone Therapy (BHT):** The hormones that the human body produces are chemically equivalent to bioidentical hormones. They might be supplied as regular prescriptions or specially formulated for each patient. There is no concrete proof that bioidentical hormones reduce the risk of breast cancer, despite the fact that they are promoted as safer or more natural substitutes for traditional hormone replacement therapy.

2. **Local HRT:** In order to treat local menopausal symptoms (such vaginal dryness), topical estrogen treatments including creams, gels, or vaginal rings are given directly to places like the vagina. Compared to systemic HRT, local HRT provides lower amounts of estrogen; so, the systemic danger, which includes the risk of breast cancer, is thought to be lower.

Oral tablets, transdermal patches, topical gels or creams, injections, and vaginal rings are some of the methods that hormone replacement therapy can provide. The risk profile can also be influenced by the mode of delivery; some research indicates that oral formulations of estrogen may be more harmful to breast health than transdermal (through the skin) distribution.

5.2. How Breast Cancer Risk Is Increased by HRT

The way hormones, especially estrogen and progesterone, affect breast tissue is the main factor influencing the association between HRT and the risk of breast cancer. Hormone-receptor-positive (ER+/PR+) breast cancer cells proliferate in response to progesterone and estrogen. HRT can promote the growth of any hormone-sensitive breast cells by raising levels of these hormones, which may hasten the onset of cancer.

HRT raises the risk of breast cancer through a number of ways, including:

- **The Function of Estrogen in Cell Proliferation:** In breast tissue, estrogen stimulates cell division. Cell development is strictly controlled in normal conditions. But when circulating estrogen levels rise either as a result of hormone replacement therapy or normal hormonal fluctuations this can cause cells to proliferate excessively, which raises the risk of mistakes in DNA replication and mutations that could start cancer. Pre-existing aberrant or precancerous cells can also benefit from estrogen's ability to promote cellular proliferation by being able to proliferate more quickly.

- **Progesterone's Effect:** Compared to estrogen-only HRT, combined HRT which contains both progesterone and estrogen—is linked to an increased risk of breast cancer. It seems that progesterone and estrogen work in concert to increase breast cell stimulation. It has been demonstrated to increase breast epithelial cell proliferation, which fosters an environment more favorable to the development of breast cancer. For this reason, women who use combined hormone replacement therapy for a longer period of time have a higher chance of developing breast cancer.

A known consequence of hormone replacement therapy, particularly combined hormone replacement therapy, is an increase in breast density. One known risk factor for breast cancer is high breast density, which is defined as the proportion of glandular or fibrous tissue to fatty tissue in the breast. In addition to raising the chance of getting cancer, dense breast tissue can cause delays in diagnosis by making tumors harder to see on mammograms.

Hormone-Receptor-Positive Tumors: An Impact
Hormone replacement treatment is more likely to have an impact on breast tumors that are either progesterone

receptor-positive (PR+) or estrogen receptor-positiv (ER+). Hormones cause these malignancies to grow, an using hormone replacement therapy (HRT) can increas exposure to estrogen and progesterone, which can promot the formation of hormone-sensitive tumors, especially ir postmenopausal women.

The longer you use HRT, the higher your chance of getting breast cancer. According to studies, women who use hormone replacement therapy for five years or longer are more likely to get breast cancer than those who use it for less time. Although it could take a few years for the risk to return to baseline, the elevated risk starts to decrease after stopping HRT.

Increased Risk with Long-Term Use: Long-term use of combined hormone replacement therapy (HRT) (estrogen plus progesterone) has been linked to a 20–30% increased risk of breast cancer compared to women who have never used HRT, according to research, including findings from the Women's Health Initiative (WHI) and other large-scale studies. A decreased but still noteworthy risk has been associated with estrogen-only HRT, especially when used for ten years or more.

Postmenopausal Breast Cancer Risk: Compared to women who do not use hormone replacement therapy, women who use it following menopause, especially after the age of 50, when natural hormone levels start to drop, are at a higher risk of developing breast cancer. Those with a family history of breast cancer or other genetic predispositions may be at a higher risk.

5.3. Recommendations for HRT Safety

Even while hormone replacement therapy (HRT) is still a useful tool for treating menopausal symptoms, especially in women whose symptoms are severe enough to negatively impact their quality of life, it's crucial to adhere to rules and procedures to reduce the risk of breast cancer. In order to balance symptom relief with safety concerns, healthcare professionals should customize HRT treatments for each patient.

Important rules for using HRT safely include:

- **Individual Risk Assessment:** Medical professional should review a woman's personal and family medical history, particularly with regard to osteoporosis, cardiovascular disease, and breast cancer, before administering hormone replacement therapy. Avoiding HRT or choosing non-hormonal options may be recommended for women with a history of breast cancer or high-risk factors (such as mutations in the BRCA gene).

- **Short-Term Use:** In order to effectively control symptoms, HRT should typically be used for the shortest amount of time and at the lowest possible dose. Many women can safely use hormone replacement therapy (HRT) to reduce menopausal symptoms for two to five years. After that, the medication should be tapered off gradually. Long-term use, particularly after age five, raises the risk of breast cancer as well as other illnesses like heart disease and stroke.

- **Type of HRT:** Depending on whether a uterus is present or not, the choice between estrogen-only and mixed HRT should be made. Estrogen-only HRT, which has a lower risk of breast cancer, is available to women without uteruses. To prevent endometrial cancer, women with an intact uterus should use combined hormone replacement therapy (HRT). However, because of the increased risk of breast cancer, the length of time they utilize combined therapy should be limited.

- **Regular Monitoring and Mammograms:** Annual mammograms and other routine breast cancer screenings should be performed on women taking hormone replacement therapy. For women who are at a higher risk, additional imaging methods like MRI may be advised because HRT can increase breast density, which may make mammograms less useful in detecting cancers.

- HRT is not a long-term treatment, so it should be reevaluated and discontinued. To find out if HRT is still required, women on the medication should have their care reviewed on a regular basis. Alternative therapy or lifestyle changes may be investigated for women who experience persistent symptoms in order to lessen their need for HRT.

- **Non-Hormonal Alternatives:** Non-hormonal methods of treating menopausal symptoms are available for women who are unable or unable to take hormone replacement therapy. These could include lifestyle changes, natural supplements, gabapentin for hot flashes, and selective serotonin reuptake inhibitors (SSRIs). These substitutes can alleviate symptoms without the cancer risks that come with hormone replacement therapy.

- **Local Hormone Therapy:** Topical estrogen therapies may be a safer option than systemic HRT for women who predominantly experience localized symptoms, such as vaginal dryness or pain. These treatments lower the risk of breast cancer by requiring little systemic absorption.

The adoption of good lifestyle practices, such as maintaining a healthy weight, exercising frequently, cutting back on alcohol, and quitting smoking, may help reduce the risk of breast cancer in women taking hormone replacement therapy. A diet high in fruits, vegetables, and whole grains can also lower the risk of cancer and promote hormone balance in general.

Although hormone replacement therapy (HRT) can greatly enhance the quality of life for women going through menopause, its usage needs to be handled carefully because it is linked to an increased risk of breast cancer. Achieving a balance between the potential health hazards and the advantages of hormone replacement therapy requires regular monitoring, personalized risk assessments, and adherence to safe usage standards. Many women can reduce their risk of breast cancer and experience relief from menopausal symptoms with cautious management.

CHAPTER 6

TREATMENT OF BREAST CANCER WITH OESTROGEN BLOCKERS

6.1. Estrogen Blockers' Mode of Action

An essential part of treating hormone-receptor-positive breast cancer is the use of estrogen blockers, sometimes referred to as anti-estrogens or estrogen antagonists. Estrogen, a hormone that stimulates the growth of many breast cancer cells, especially those that are estrogen receptor-positive (ER+), is inhibited by these medications. To fully appreciate estrogen blockers' function in the treatment of breast cancer, one must comprehend their mechanism of action.

Estrogen blockers primarily work by either reducing the body's levels of estrogen or by blocking the hormone's ability to connect to its receptors. As a result, cancer cells are deprived of the stimulation they need to develop and multiply. There are two primary types of estrogen blockers:

1. **Selective Estrogen Receptor Modulators (SERMs):** Tamoxifen and other medications bind to the estrogen receptors on breast cancer cells to prevent the attachment of estrogen. While SERMs may let estrogen to operate normally in other regions of the body (such as the bones), they block the proliferative effect of estrogen on breast tissue by occupying the receptor sites. SERMs are particularly helpful in the treatment of breast cancer because of their selective activity.

2. **Aromatase Inhibitors (AIs):** AIs, like anastrozole, function by reducing the body's total estrogen levels. The main source of estrogen in postmenopausal women is the enzyme aromatase, which is found in adipose tissue and converts androgens into estrogen. Aromatase inhibitors prevent this conversion, which lowers blood estrogen levels and, as a result, lessens the activation of cancer cells. Since postmenopausal women's ovarian estrogen production has already stopped, these medications work especially well for them.

By preventing estrogen's ability to encourage the formation of cancer, SERMs and AIs both significantly lower the chance of breast cancer recurrence. The particulars of the tumor and the patient's menopausal state have a significant impact on how effective they are.

6.2. Tamoxifen: An ER+ Breast Cancer Standard Treatment

One of the most well-known and often used estrogen blockers for the treatment of breast cancer, especially ER+ breast cancer, is tamoxifen. For many years, it has been a mainstay of hormone therapy for breast cancer and is a member of the class of medications known as Selective Estrogen Receptor Modulators (SERMs).

- **The Way Tamoxifen Operates:** By attaching itself to the estrogen receptors on breast cancer cells, tamoxifen stops estrogen from triggering the growth signals of the cells. Tamoxifen does not totally inhibit the generation or action of estrogen in other areas of the body, but it does prevent the effects of estrogen in breast tissue. Actually, tamoxifen can function as a partial estrogen agonist in some organs, such as the heart and bones, providing some protection against heart disease and osteoporosis.

- **Clinical Use of Tamoxifen:** Tamoxifen is mainly used to treat ER+ breast cancer in premenopausal and postmenopausal women as an adjuvant (post-surgery) and neoadjuvant (pre-surgery) treatment. Depending on the patient's risk factors and reaction to treatment, it is usually given for five to ten years. In certain situations, it might be used to shield high-risk women against breast cancer.

- **Benefits and Efficacy:** Studies have repeatedly demonstrated that tamoxifen increases overall survival rates for women with hormone-receptor-positive breast cancer and lowers the chance of breast cancer recurrence. Tamoxifen also lowers the risk of developing contralateral breast cancer, which is cancer of the opposite breast, by inhibiting the effects of estrogen. Tamoxifen is a staple in breast cancer treatment regimens around the world due to its long-term effectiveness in avoiding recurrence.

- **Risks and Side Effects:** Tamoxifen has side effects, just like any other medicine. Menopausal symptoms include mood swings, vaginal dryness, and hot flashes are among the frequent adverse effects. Blood clots (pulmonary embolism and deep vein thrombosis) and uterine cancer are two more severe hazards linked to tamoxifen. Even though these hazards are uncommon, they must be considered in relation to the substantial advantages of tamoxifen in lowering the recurrence of breast cancer.

- **Preventing Breast Cancer in Women at High Risk:** Tamoxifen is authorized to lower the risk of breast cancer in women who are at high risk because of genetic factors, family history, or other predispositions, in addition to its use in active breast cancer treatment. Tamoxifen is an effective cancer prevention medication that has been proved in clinical trials to lower the incidence of breast cancer in high-risk women by as much as 50%.

6.3. Novel Treatments for Estrogen Blocking

Even though tamoxifen and aromatase inhibitors have long been known to be successful treatments for ER+ breast cancer, research into novel estrogen-blocking medicines is still continuing. These developments seek to enhance results, lessen adverse effects, and offer more individualized therapy choices depending on the biology and genetics of each tumor.

- **Aromatase Inhibitors (AIs):** Letrozole and exemestane are two examples of AIs that have transformed the way postmenopausal women with ER+ breast cancer are treated. As previously stated, AIs successfully reduce estrogen levels in postmenopausal women by inhibiting the aromatase enzyme. Although some postmenopausal women continue to take tamoxifen, AIs are becoming more and more popular because of their superior ability to lower the risk of cancer recurrence. According to research, AIs can lower postmenopausal women's risk of breast cancer recurrence by roughly 30% more than tamoxifen. To increase patient compliance and lessen adverse effects such bone density loss, new AI formulations and delivery systems are being researched.

- **SERDs, or selective estrogen receptor downregulators:** SERDs are a more recent class of medications that function by both blocking and degrading estrogen receptors. For instance, fulvestrant inhibits the cancer cell's ability to respond to estrogen by binding to the estrogen receptor and encouraging its death. Fulvestrant has demonstrated potential in the treatment of metastatic breast cancer and cancers that have developed resistance to aromatase inhibitors or tamoxifen. Researchers are looking into the possibility of oral SERDs, which would provide a more practical and patient-friendly option than the injectable variants that are already on the market.

- **Inhibitors of CDK4/6:** CDK4/6 inhibitors, such as palbociclib, ribociclib, and abemaciclib, have become a significant adjunct to hormone therapy for ER+ breast cancer, despite not being an estrogen blocker. These medications impede the growth of cancer cells by blocking cyclin-dependent kinases 4 and 6, two proteins involved in cell division. Women with advanced or metastatic breast cancer have demonstrated notable gains in progression-free survival when using CDK4/6 inhibitors in conjunction with aromatase inhibitors or fulvestrant. Particularly for patients whose cancer has advanced after receiving early hormone therapy, this class of medications marks a significant leap in hormone-based treatments.

- **AIs and Next-Generation SERMs:** Next-generation AIs and SERMs with better efficacy and fewer negative effects are being developed by researchers. These more recent medications are made to target estrogen receptors more specifically, which may lower the risk of tamoxifen-related blood clots and uterine cancer. Furthermore, customized therapies that are adapted to each patient's unique tumor profile are now possible thanks to developments in our understanding of the molecular pathways underlying breast cancer.

- **Targeted Hormone Therapies:** As precision medicine advances, hormone treatments are becoming increasingly customized according to a patient's genetic composition and tumor features. More advanced methods for identifying which patients may benefit most from estrogen-blocking medications may result from ongoing research into the genetic and molecular causes of breast cancer. To anticipate medication response, reduce resistance, and provide more individualized treatment plans, new biomarkers and genetic testing are being developed.

- **Combination medicines:** Combination medicines represent another development in estrogen-blocking drugs. Researchers hope to improve therapy efficacy and circumvent resistance mechanisms that emerge over time by combining estrogen blockers with other targeted medicines, such as immune checkpoint inhibitors or PARP inhibitors. Clinical trials are demonstrating the potential of these combination approaches, especially for individuals with metastatic or advanced breast cancer.

Estrogen blockers have a fundamental and developing function in the treatment of breast cancer. New treatments and combinations are being created as research progresses, giving patients with ER+ breast cancer hope for better results, a higher quality of life, and more specialized care. Patients and healthcare professionals can collaborate to make well-informed decisions on the management of breast cancer by being aware of the mechanisms of action, the effectiveness of current treatments, such as tamoxifen, and the exciting prospects for novel therapies.

CHAPTER 7

THE FUNCTION OF AROMATASE INHIBITORS IN BREAST CANCER

7.1. Aromatase Inhibitors: What Are They?

A family of medications known as aromatase inhibitors (AIs) is mostly used to treat postmenopausal women with hormone receptor-positive breast cancer. These drugs function by blocking the enzyme aromatase, which is in charge of changing androgens which are made in the adrenal glands into estrogens. Reducing estrogen is a crucial therapy technique for breast cancer since it can stimulate the proliferation of hormone receptor-positive (ER+) breast cancer cells.

At the moment, three main aromatase inhibitors are in use:

1. One of the most often prescribed AIs, anastrozole (Arimidex) is used to treat breast cancer in both its

early and late stages.

2. **Letrozole (Femara):** Also used extensively to lower the chance of cancer recurrence, particularly in postmenopausal women.

3. **Aromasin (Exemestane):** Exemestane, a steroidal AI with a structurally distinct structure from anastrozole and letrozole, binds to the aromatase enzymc irreversibly, rendering it permanently inactive.

Because the ovaries stop releasing large levels of estrogen after menopause and the hormone is mostly produced in peripheral tissues via the aromatase route, AIs are more effective in postmenopausal women. When this route is blocked, ER+ breast cancer cells are deprived of the estrogen necessary for growth and division.

7.2. Aromatase's Function in Postmenopausal Estrogen Production

The ovaries are the primary source of estrogen in premenopausal women. However, as ovarian function deteriorates after menopause, the body's estrogen levels sharply drop. In spite of this, the aromatase enzyme still produces trace levels of estrogen in peripheral tissues such as muscle, fat, and the adrenal glands. Androgens, such as testosterone and androstenedione, are changed into estrogen via aromatase.

Despite having lower levels than in premenopausal women, postmenopausal estrogen production is adequate to promote the proliferation of ER+ breast cancer cells. The following is the mechanism:

1. **Enzyme aromatase:** Adipose (fat) tissue is one of the tissues that contains aromatase, which catalyzes the transformation of androgens into estrogen.

2. **Peripheral estrogen production:** This pathway becomes the main source of estrogen in the bloodstream in postmenopausal women.

3. **Tumors' local production of estrogen:** Higher aromatase concentrations in some breast cancer tissues can enable localized estrogen synthesis, which can promote tumor growth even in the presence of low systemic estrogen levels.

By blocking this transformation of androgens into

estrogen, aromatase inhibitors function. By doing this, they successfully lower the amount of estrogen in the blood and lessen its impact on breast cancer cells. As a result, AIs are a vital tool for treating postmenopausal women with ER+ breast cancer.

7.3. A Comparison of Oestrogen Blockers and Aromatase Inhibitors

Although ER+ breast cancer is treated with both aromatase inhibitors (AIs) and estrogen blockers (like tamoxifen), their target patient populations and modes of action are different. Healthcare providers can make well-informed treatment options depending on the patient's menopausal status, tumor features, and personal risk factors by being aware of these distinctions.

Aromatase Inhibitors:

Mechanism of Action: By blocking the aromatase enzyme, which converts androgens into estrogen, AIs reduce systemic estrogen levels. Because postmenopausal women manufacture the majority of their estrogen in peripheral tissues rather than the ovaries, they are mostly used in these women.

- Tamoxifen and other SERMs are examples of estrogen blockers. Tamoxifen functions by attaching itself to breast cancer cells' estrogen receptors and blocking the activation of these receptors by estrogen. It inhibits the hormone's capacity to promote the formation of cancer cells in breast tissue rather than lowering the body's total estrogen levels.

Patient Population:

- **Aromatase Inhibitors:** AIs work best in postmenopausal women whose aromatase activity serves as their main source of estrogen. Because the ovaries continue to produce large amounts of estrogen, AIs are usually ineffective in premenopausal women unless used in conjunction with ovarian suppression.

- **Tamoxifen, an estrogen blocker:** Both premenopausal and postmenopausal women can use tamoxifen. Because it competes with estrogen for receptor binding without lowering systemic estrogen levels, which can be advantageous for bone health and other physiological processes, it continues to be the standard of therapy for premenopausal women.

Efficacy in Various Stages:

- **Aromatase Inhibitors:** Research has indicated that AIs may offer a better risk reduction for breast cancer recurrence than tamoxifen, particularly for postmenopausal women. Clinical trials, for instance, have shown that women who receive AI treatment are less likely to experience a cancer recurrence, especially while the malignancy is still in its early stages.

- **Tamoxifen**: In postmenopausal women, tamoxifen may not have the same impact on recurrence rates as AIs, despite its continued high effectiveness. It is still a viable choice, though, especially for women who are unable to handle the negative impacts of AIs.

Adverse Effects:

- **Aromatase Inhibitors:** Joint discomfort, hot flushes, exhaustion, and bone weakening (osteopenia or osteoporosis) are typical adverse effects of AIs. Women may be more susceptible to fractures as a result of a decrease in bone mineral density brought on by a drop in estrogen levels. Therefore, for patients receiving long-term AI medication, bone density monitoring is frequently advised.

- **Tamoxifen:** Hot flashes, dry vagina, and an elevated risk of blood clots and uterine cancer are among the adverse effects of tamoxifen. Tamoxifen is a better choice for people who are at risk of osteoporosis, though, because it can protect bone density in postmenopausal women.

Duration of Treatment:

- **Aromatase Inhibitors:** AIs are usually recommended for 5–10 years, either as a primary treatment or in a sequential method called as "switch therapy," which involves taking tamoxifen for two to three years. It has been demonstrated that this strategy lowers recurrence rates and increases overall survival.

- Similar to AIs, tamoxifen is typically taken for a period of five to ten years. After a few years of treatment, some patients, especially postmenopausal women may move from tamoxifen to an AI in order to further lower the chance of recurrence.

Risk of Cancer Recurrence: Research has shown that AIs significantly lower the risk of breast cancer recurrence in postmenopausal women compared to tamoxifen. Tamoxifen is still very successful for premenopausal women, nevertheless, and ovarian suppression combined with AIs is becoming more and more popular as a substitute therapy approach.

Aromatase inhibitors are essential for treating ER+ breast cancer, especially in women who have gone through menopause. Their use must be carefully considered against potential adverse effects such bone loss and joint discomfort, even though they offer significant benefits in boosting survival rates and lowering the chance of cancer recurrence. Healthcare professionals must weigh the patient's menopausal status, general health, and personal risk factors when evaluating AIs against estrogen blockers like tamoxifen in order to choose the best course of action.

CHAPTER 8

LIFESTYLE AND ENVIRONMENTAL ASPECTS AFFECTING

ESTROGEN LEVELS

It's crucial to comprehend how lifestyle and environmental factors affect estrogen levels, especially when it comes to breast cancer. Higher amounts of circulating estrogen can promote tumor growth in estrogen receptor-positive (ER+) breast cancers, where estrogen plays a key role in the genesis of the disease. This chapter examines the main environmental and lifestyle factors that affect the synthesis and metabolism of estrogen and raise the risk of breast cancer, including nutrition, obesity, and environmental pollutants.

8.1. Diet and How It Affects Oestrogen Production

The body's levels of hormones, especially estrogen, are greatly influenced by diet. The risk of breast cancer can be influenced by the increase or reduction of estrogen levels caused by specific foods, nutrients, and dietary habits. The following are some dietary components that impact estrogen levels:

Plant-based substances that structurally resemble estrogen are known as phytoestrogens. Phytoestrogens, which can imitate estrogen in the body but function far less strongly than the body's natural estrogen, are present in foods like soybeans, flaxseeds, lentils, and whole grains. High phytoestrogen intake may lower the risk of breast cancer by preventing stronger estrogens from attaching to estrogen receptors, according to some research, but other studies express worries about the possibility that phytoestrogens could promote estrogen-dependent tumor growth. Individual hormone sensitivity, the type of breast cancer, and the quantity of phytoestrogens ingested all seem to have an impact.

- **Dietary Fat Intake:** Research has indicated that diets rich in saturated fats, which are frequently included in processed foods, red meat, and some dairy products, are linked to increased levels of estrogen in the blood. On the other hand, diets high in good fats, such omega-3 fatty acids from nuts seeds, and fish, may reduce estrogen levels and prevent breast cancer. These good fats may help maintain balanced hormone synthesis, lower inflammation, and increase insulin sensitivity.

- **Fiber:** By binding excess estrogen in the gut and promoting its elimination through the digestive system, a high-fiber diet, especially one that includes fruits, vegetables, and whole grains, can help reduce estrogen levels. A lower incidence of ER+ breast cancer has also been linked to increased fiber consumption. Additionally, fiber affects gut bacteria, which may be involved in the control and metabolism of estrogen.

- **Alcohol Consumption:** Alcohol has been demonstrated to increase estrogen levels by obstructing the liver's effective metabolization of the hormone. Because it raises the amount of estrogen in the blood, regular alcohol use, especially excessive drinking, is associated with a higher risk of breast cancer. Furthermore, alcohol may raise the risk of breast cancer by producing reactive oxygen species (ROS), which can damage DNA and encourage the growth of tumors.

- **Cruciferous Vegetables:** Broccoli, cauliflower, kale, and Brussels sprouts are among the vegetables that contain indole-3-carbinol, a substance that supports the metabolism of estrogen and lowers the levels of potentially hazardous estrogen metabolites. These substances may reduce the risk of breast cancer by encouraging the synthesis of less powerful versions of estrogen.

In conclusion, nutrition has a significant impact on estrogen levels. Lowering estrogen levels and lowering the risk of breast cancer may be achieved by eating a diet high in phytoestrogens, fiber, healthy fats, and cruciferous vegetables and low in alcohol and saturated fat.

8.2. Obesity and Elevated Production of Oestrogen

One known risk factor for breast cancer, especially in postmenopausal women, is obesity. The connection between estrogen production and adipose (fat) tissue is the main cause of this association. Fat tissue becomes the main source of estrogen through the aromatization of androgens during menopause, when the ovaries cease to produce appreciable levels of the hormone.

- **Adipose Tissue and Aromatase Activity:** The enzyme aromatase, which is found in fat tissue, is responsible for the conversion of androgens (like testosterone) into estrogen. Because obese people have more adipose tissue, their aromatase activity is higher, which increases the quantity of estrogen they produce. ER+ breast tumors may grow more quickly as a result of this increased estrogen level.

- **Chronic Inflammation:** Low-grade chronic inflammation is linked to obesity and can increase the risk of breast cancer. Growth factors and cytokines are released when inflammation occurs, and this may stimulate aromatase activity and raise estrogen levels. Furthermore, by damaging DNA and encouraging tumor angiogenesis the growth of new blood vessels that supply the tumor with nutrients inflammation can provide a microenvironment that aids in the advancement of cancer.

- **Estrogen Levels and Insulin Resistance:** Insulin resistance and hyperinsulinemia, or elevated levels of circulating insulin, are frequently caused by obesity. Because insulin stimulates the synthesis of sex hormone-binding globulin (SHBG), a protein that binds to estrogen and decreases its bioavailability, elevated insulin levels are linked to increased estrogen production. More free (active) estrogen is available to promote the formation of breast tissue when SHBG levels are low.

- **Impact on the Outcomes of Breast Cancer:** Obesity not only increases the incidence of breast cancer but also has been associated with worse outcomes for women who have been diagnosed with the disease. Compared to their lean counterparts, obese women typically have larger tumors, higher metastasis rates, and shorter survival rates. Both the elevated estrogen levels and the inflammatory milieu brought on by obesity are responsible for this.

A key tactic for lowering estrogen levels and the risk o breast cancer, especially in postmenopausal women, i weight management by diet, exercise, and lifestyle modifications.

8.3. Estrogen Disruption and Environmental Toxins

Endocrine-disrupting chemicals (EDCs) are a class of environmental pollutants that can disrupt the body's hormonal systems, especially by imitating or inhibiting estrogen. Because of their capacity to bind to estrogen receptors and stimulate aberrant cell growth, these substances often referred to as xenoestrogens—have been connected to an increased risk of breast cancer.

Typical Xenoestrogens:

1. **Bisphenol A (BPA):** This chemical, which is included in plastic items, food can linings, and receipts, can mimic estrogen in the body. According to studies, BPA exposure can accelerate the growth of breast cancer cells, particularly in ER+ breast cancer.

2. **Phthalates:** Found in plasticizers, cosmetics, and personal care items, phthalates have been connected to hormonal abnormalities, such as high estrogen levels, and can interfere with the endocrine system.

3. **Pesticides:** Some pesticides have estrogenic effects, including DDT and its metabolites. These chemicals are persistent in the environment and can build up in the food chain, exposing humans even though they are prohibited in many countries.

4. **Parabens:** Preservatives with mild estrogenic action, parabens are present in a lot of cosmetics and personal care items. Research indicates that prolonged exposure to parabens may raise the risk of hormone-dependent malignancies, while their impact on breast cancer risk is still up for debate.

Hormone Disruption Mechanisms: By attaching to cell estrogen receptors, xenoestrogens replicate the effects of natural estrogen. These substances can have cumulative effects even though they are frequently less potent than the body's natural estrogen. Multiple EDC exposure over time can increase estrogenic activity in breast tissue, raising the possibility of malignant transformation and cell proliferation.

Cutting Down on Exposure: One crucial preventive measure is to limit exposure to xenoestrogens. Among the suggestions are:

- Steer clear of plastic containers while storing food particularly when heating it.
- Selecting BPA-free goods and utilizing containers made of glass or stainless steel.
- Minimizing the use of personal care and cosmetics that contain parabens and phthalates.
- Organic food should be prioritized in order to reduce exposure to pesticide residues.

Public Health and Research Issues: The complete effect of xenoestrogens on the risk of breast cancer is still being investigated. More public knowledge of the possible health concerns associated with EDCs and more regulations on their use in consumer products are demands made by a number of scientists and public health organizations.

Estrogen levels and the risk of breast cancer are significantly influenced by lifestyle and environmental factors. The risk of hormone receptor-positive breast cancer can be increased by diet, obesity, and exposure to environmental pollutants, all of which can increase estrogen production or mimic its effects. People can take proactive measures to lower their estrogen levels and reduce their risk of breast cancer by addressing these factors through dietary modifications, weight control, and limiting exposure to endocrine-disrupting substances.

CHAPTER 9

STRATEGIES TO PREVENT BREAST CANCER CAUSED BY
OESTROGEN

Although there are several risk factors for breast cancer, estrogen is crucial to the initiation and spread of hormone receptor-positive (HR+) breast cancers. A multimodal strategy that incorporates early detection, hormonal treatments, and lifestyle modifications is needed to prevent estrogen-driven breast cancer. In order to lower the risk of breast cancer by treating its hormonal foundations, this chapter explores important prevention measures.

9.1. The Significance of Prompt Identification in Cancers Associated with Oestrogen

A key component of preventing breast cancer, particularly estrogen-driven tumors, is early identification. Compared to other types of breast cancer, estrogen receptor-positive (ER+) breast tumors often grow more slowly, therefore early diagnosis is a very effective way to increase survival rates and lower morbidity.

- Mammograms continue to be the gold standard for screening for breast cancer, particularly when it comes to identifying small, early-stage tumors that may not be perceptible during physical examinations. Regular mammography screening can lower the death rate from breast cancer by identifying the disease at an earlier, more manageable stage, according to studies. Regular mammograms are advised for women over 50 or those who are at high risk because of hormonal or hereditary causes.

- **Magnetic Resonance Imaging (MRI):** MRI may be used in conjunction with mammography for women who are more susceptible to estrogen-driven breast cancer, such as those who have a family history of the disease or who have known mutations in genes like BRCA1 or BRCA2. Because MRI is more sensitive, it can identify malignancies that mammograms would overlook, especially in women with thick breast tissue.

- **Genetic Testing:** Genetic testing can detect abnormalities in genes including BRCA1, BRCA2 and PALB2 linked to an elevated risk of breast cancer in people with a family history of the disease. Early detection of these mutations enables more individualized screening procedures and prophylactic surgeries, chemoprevention, or improved surveillance.

- Although it is not frequently employed in breast cancer screening, tracking circulating estrogen levels can reveal information about a person's risk of developing breast cancer, especially in postmenopausal women or those receiving hormone replacement therapy (HRT). One established risk factor for the emergence of ER+ breast tumors is elevated estrogen levels.

- **Clinical Exams and Breast Self-Examinations:** Even while clinical breast exams (CBE) and breast self-examinations (BSE) are no longer regarded as primary screening procedures, they still contribute to early diagnosis, especially when paired with imaging modalities. BSE helps women learn how their breasts should feel and appear, which makes it simpler to spot alterations. Healthcare professionals can use CBE to find anomalies that could need more research.

9.2: Does Prophylactic Oestrogen Suppression Work?

One aggressive preventative measure to lower the incidence of breast cancer in high-risk patients is prophylactic estrogen suppression. This strategy entails lowering the body's estrogen levels through medication or surgery, which lessens the activation of ER+ breast cells.

- **SERMs, or selective estrogen receptor modulators:** In high-risk women, medications such as raloxifene and tamoxifen are frequently used to prevent breast cancer. These SERMs lower the risk of estrogen-stimulated cell proliferation by preventing estrogen from attaching to its receptors in breast tissue. According to clinical studies, tamoxifen can lower a woman's risk of ER+ breast cancer by as much as 50% if she has a high risk of the disease. The advantages of SERMs must be balanced against their drawbacks, which include hot flashes, an elevated risk of blood clots, and uterine cancer.

- **Aromatase Inhibitors (AIs):** Aromatase inhibitors, such letrozole or anastrozole, may help postmenopausal women who are at high risk of breast cancer. AIs function by blocking the enzyme aromatase, which is in charge of postmenopausal women's conversion of androgens into estrogen. AIs can dramatically minimize the risk of ER+ breast cancer by reducing systemic estrogen levels. Although adverse effects including joint pain and bone density loss can happen, clinical research has shown that postmenopausal women taking AIs have a 50–60% lower incidence of breast cancer.

- **The surgical removal of the ovaries, or oophorectomy:** Prophylactic oophorectomy may be explored in premenopausal women who have a markedly increased risk of breast cancer, such as those who have BRCA mutations. The likelihood of getting ER+ breast cancer is decreased by removing the ovaries, which significantly reduces estrogen production. Despite being quite successful, oophorectomy causes early menopause and all of its symptoms, such as mood swings, hot flashes, and an elevated risk of cardiovascular disease and osteoporosis. When deciding whether to have this operation, the patient's risk profile and quality of life must be carefully taken into account.

- **hazards and Considerations:** Although estrogen suppression can effectively lower the risk of breast cancer, there are hazards associated with it. Significant adverse effects, such as bone loss, cardiovascular risks, and a reduction in general quality of life, can result from prolonged estrogen deficiency. A person's age, risk factors, general health, and personal preferences must all be considered when deciding whether to undertake prophylactic estrogen suppression.

9.3 Changes in Lifestyle to Reduce Estrogen Levels

By lowering the body's estrogen levels, lifestyle changes can be a very effective way to minimize the risk of breast cancer. These adjustments not only enhance general health but also focus on important variables that affect the synthesis and metabolism of estrogen.

- **Maintaining a Healthy Weight:** As was covered in earlier chapters, aromatase activity in adipose tissue (fat) is a primary source of estrogen production during menopause. Breast cancer risk can be decreased and excess estrogen levels can be decreased by maintaining a healthy weight through regular exercise and a balanced diet. Research indicates that while women who keep a steady, healthy weight lower their risk of developing postmenopausal breast cancer, those who gain a substantial amount of weight during adulthood have a higher risk.

- Regular exercise has been demonstrated to promote

hormone balance and reduce circulating estrogen levels. Exercise maintains a healthy estrogen metabolism, lowers insulin resistance, and reduces body fat. Regular exercise also lowers inflammation and strengthens the immune system, both of which help prevent cancer. In addition to muscle-strengthening exercises, guidelines suggest engaging in at least 150 minutes of moderate-intensity aerobic exercise or 75 minutes of vigorous-intensity exercise per week.

- **Dietary Choices:** By promoting the excretion of excess estrogen through the digestive tract, a plant-based diet high in fiber, whole grains, fruits, and vegetables can support a balanced estrogen metabolism. Compounds in certain meals, such cruciferous vegetables (broccoli, kale, and Brussels sprouts), aid in the detoxification of estrogen and encourage the synthesis of advantageous estrogen metabolites.

Because they function as weak oestrogens and may prevent the more powerful effects of natural estrogen, phytoestrogens, which are present in soy products, flaxseeds, and legumes, may also have a preventive impact against breast cancer.

- **Restricting Alcohol:** Regular alcohol use is connected to an increased risk of breast cancer, and alcohol consumption is linked to an increase in estrogen levels. This risk can be decreased by consuming no more than one drink of alcohol every day or by abstaining from it completely.

- **Minimizing Endocrine-Disrupting Chemical (EDC) Exposure:** Bisphenol A (BPA), phthalates, and certain pesticides are examples of environmental pollutants that can mimic estrogen in the body and cause hormonal abnormalities. The risk of breast cancer may be decreased by limiting exposure to certain substances.

When storing and heating food, choose glass or stainless steel containers rather than plastic ones.

- To prevent pesticide residues, use organic vegetables.
- Steer clear of personal care items that contain

phthalates and parabens, which are frequently found in cosmetics.

Managing Stress: Prolonged stress has been demonstrated to throw off the balance of hormones, leading to elevated cortisol levels, which can have an indirect impact on the production of estrogen. Stress-reduction methods including yoga, meditation, mindfulness, and deep breathing exercises can help control hormone levels and enhance general health.

Preventing estrogen-driven breast cancer necessitates a multifaceted strategy that includes lifestyle changes, hormonal therapies, and early identification. Estrogen suppression treatments offer tailored prevention for high-risk patients, while routine screening and early risk factor identification enable prompt intervention. Changes in lifestyle that lower the risk of cancer and support healthy hormone levels are equally significant. It is feasible to considerably reduce the risk of estrogen-related breast cancer and enhance long-term health outcomes by combining lifestyle and medicinal interventions.

CHAPTER 10

RESEARCH ON BREAST CANCER AND OESTROGEN TARGETING IN THE FUTURE

The function of estrogen and its receptor pathways remains a major focus of breast cancer research, especially in the creation of tailored and targeted medicines. We are now entering a new era of estrogen receptor-positive (ER+) breast cancer treatments that are getting more sophisticated, with the possibility for more efficient and customized approaches because of developments in genetic research, molecular biology, and precision medicine. The future of breast cancer research is examined in this chapter, with particular attention paid to advancements in ER+ treatments, genetic discoveries, and customized treatment plans that could lead to better outcomes in the management of breast cancer.

10.1. Advances in ER+ Breast Cancer Targeted Therapies

Estrogen drives the growth of ER+ breast cancers, which make up about 70% of all occurrences of breast cancer. Treatment for breast cancer has therefore relied heavily on treatments that either directly target estrogen receptors or interfere with estrogen signaling pathways. New developments are expanding the use of conventional hormone treatments, resulting in more advanced and non-toxic methods.

SERDs, or selective estrogen receptor degraders: Conventional treatments, such as tamoxifen, inhibit the estrogen receptor by acting as Selective Estrogen Receptor Modulators (SERMs). But by encouraging the breakdown and downregulation of estrogen receptors, new treatments called Selective Estrogen Receptor Degraders (SERDs) go one step further. New oral SERDs are being developed, however fulvestrant is one such SERD that is currently in clinical usage. These medications might be superior to current treatments, particularly for patients who have grown resistant to aromatase inhibitors or SERMs.

Inhibitors of CDK4/6: The use of cyclin-dependent kinase 4/6 (CDK4/6) inhibitors, such as palbociclib, ribociclib, and abemaciclib, is another significant development in the treatment of ER+ breast cancer. The way these medications function is by blocking the CDK4/6 enzymes, which are essential for cell division. These inhibitors stop the cancer cells' cell cycle, which stops the growth and spread of tumors. When used with hormonal treatments such as fulvestrant or aromatase inhibitors, CDK4/6 inhibitors have been demonstrated to dramatically increase progression-free survival in patients with advanced ER+ breast cancer.

Inhibitors of the PI3K/AKT/mTOR Pathway: The PI3K/AKT/mTOR signaling pathway is dysregulated in many ER+ breast tumors, which encourages cancer cell survival and treatment resistance. One promising approach to treating breast cancer that is resistant to hormone therapy is to target this route. The approval of medications such as alpelisib (a PI3K inhibitor) and everolimus (an mTOR inhibitor) for use in conjunction with hormone therapy has given patients whose malignancies have advanced in spite of conventional treatments additional options.

ADCs, or antibody-drug conjugates, are: An innovative method of treating cancer, antibody-drug conjugates combine the strong cytotoxicity of chemotherapeutic drugs with the specificity of monoclonal antibodies. ADCs can deliver a chemotherapeutic medication directly to cancer cells while preserving healthy tissues by attaching a monoclonal antibody that targets the estrogen receptor or other cancer-related proteins. This focused strategy improves treatment efficacy while lowering systemic toxicity. Trastuzumab deruxtecan is one such ADC that has demonstrated potential in HER2+ breast cancer, and comparable strategies are being investigated for ER+ subtypes.

The use of combination therapy, which targets several pathways at once, is growing in popularity as our knowledge of the biology of breast cancer expands. For example, in ER+ breast cancer, combining CDK4/6 inhibitors with PI3K or SERD inhibitors can address several resistance pathways. Personalized combinations of targeted drugs that have more long-lasting effects with fewer side effects may become more and more important in the treatment of breast cancer in the future.

10.2. Genetic Studies of Mutations in Estrogen Receptors

Our knowledge of breast cancer has been completely transformed by genetic research, especially in the identification of mutations that affect the cancers' response to hormone and estrogen treatments. Finding mutations in the estrogen receptor gene (ESR1), which can lead to resistance to traditional hormonal treatments, has been one of the most important discoveries in recent years.

ESR1 Mutations and Therapy Resistance: The estrogen receptor can become constitutively active even when estrogen is not present due to structural changes caused by mutations in the ESR1 gene. This makes it possible for cancer cells to proliferate in spite of therapies intended to prevent the generation of estrogen or the activation of receptors. Patients with metastatic ER+ breast cancer who have received aromatase inhibitor treatment are most likely to have ESR1 mutations. It is essential to comprehend the frequency and consequences of ESR1 mutations in order to create novel treatments that can circumvent this resistance mechanism.

Detection of Mutations via Liquid Biopsies: The use of liquid biopsies to identify ESR1 mutations and other genetic changes is one of the most intriguing uses of genetic research in breast cancer. Through the analysis of circulating tumor DNA (ctDNA) in the bloodstream, liquid biopsies provide a non-invasive means of tracking the progression of tumors and instantly detecting alterations. By using this method, resistance mutations can be found early on, allowing doctors to modify treatment plans before the cancer spreads. Future individualized breast cancer treatment is anticipated to heavily rely on liquid biopsies.

In addition to ESR1 mutations, scientists are discovering additional genetic changes that impact estrogen receptor signaling and the development of breast cancer. For instance, the function of epigenetic modifications that control gene expression and mutations in genes implicated in the PI3K/AKT/mTOR pathway in ER+ breast cancer is being studied. It will be easier to improve treatment plans and create new treatments that target the entire range of genetic alterations that cause estrogen receptor activation.

10.3. Oestrogen Profile-Based Customized Treatment Plans

Breast cancer is not an exception to the trend of personalized medicine becoming the new norm in cancer therapy. Clinicians can optimize treatment success and minimize side effects by customizing medicines to the unique molecular and genetic features of each patient's tumor. Based on a person's estrogen profile, which includes receptor status, the existence of mutations, and general hormone metabolism, tailored treatments for ER+ breast cancer are being developed.

Future treatment choices will be guided by a thorough assessment of a patient's estrogen receptor status, which includes the presence of ESR1 mutations, the co-expression of other hormone receptors (like progesterone receptors), and the activity of downstream signaling pathways. This might entail molecular diagnostic studies that offer a thorough understanding of the tumor's hormone reliance, enabling medical professionals to select the best hormonal or targeted treatments.

- **Predictive Biomarkers:** Biomarkers are crucial instruments for forecasting a tumor's reaction to particular treatments. Biomarkers such as the progesterone receptor (PR) status and Ki-67, a measure of cell proliferation, are already utilized in ER+ breast cancer to help predict how well the disease will respond to hormonal treatments. In order to improve outcomes through more individualized care, future research attempts to find other biomarkers that can more precisely predict therapy resistance or responsiveness to novel treatments.

- **Tailored Drug Combinations:** To target various facets of tumor biology, personalized therapy approaches sometimes entail mixing several medications. A PI3K inhibitor may be necessary in addition to normal hormone therapy for a patient with a PI3K mutation, while a combination of a

SERD and a CDK4/6 inhibitor may be beneficial for a patient with a high tumor burden and a discovered ESR1 mutation. The capacity to tailor treatment according to each patient's own tumor profile will advance with the development of novel targeted medicines, providing more robust and efficient results.

- **Approaches to Adaptive Treatment:** Adaptive treatment approaches that alter as the cancer does are another aspect of individualized cancer care in the future. Clinicians will be able to modify therapies in response to new resistance mutations or modifications in the tumor's genetic profile through routine monitoring with liquid biopsies and other cutting-edge diagnostic techniques. This dynamic method of treatment offers a more tailored and responsive approach to controlling ER+ breast cancer by guaranteeing that medicines continue to be effective throughout the course of the disease.

In conclusion, with developments in targeted medicines, genetic studies, and the creation of individualized treatment plans, the future of estrogen targeting and breast cancer research is bright. With more potent and less harmful treatment options, these advancements could greatly enhance outcomes for individuals with ER+ breast cancer. There is significant promise for advancements in the prevention, diagnosis, and treatment of this common and complicated condition over the next 10 years as our knowledge of estrogen receptor biology continues to grow.

ABOUT THE AUTHOR

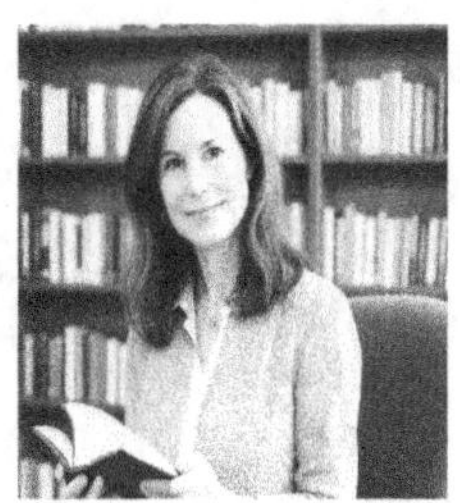

Sophia Royce Smartwell is a committed writer who specializes in wellness and health, offering insightful information on mental and physical health. She is deeply passionate about educating readers on important health issues and trying to close the knowledge gap between medical research and common sense. Her publications are designed to give people the knowledge they need to take charge of their health in an understandable, approachable, and evidence-based manner.

www.ingramcontent.com/pod-product-compliance
Lightning Source LLC
Chambersburg PA
CBHW050803250726
48653CB00006B/2043